RENAL DIET
COOKBOOK
BREAKFAST RECIPES

HEALTHY RECIPES WITH LOW POTASSIUM,
LOW SODIUM AND LOW PHOSPHORUS TO STOP
KIDNEY DISEASE AND AVOID DIALYSIS

CONTENTS

INTRODUCTION

ndividuals with deteriorating kidneys must stick to a renal or kidney diet to lessen up the measure of waste in their blood. These wastes in the blood are the results of diets and liquids that are devoured. When the kidneys aren't performing well, they don't tackle or evacuate waste appropriately and precisely. If that waste remains or is left stuck in the blood, it can adversely influence a patient's electrolyte measures. Following a kidney diet may help advance kidney function and slow the complete kidney failure or dysfunction movement.

A diet is assumed as a renal diet if it lacks sodium, phosphorous, and protein. A renal diet likewise underlines the significance of consuming top-notch protein and restricting the consumption of liquids. A few patients may also need to limit potassium and calcium. Each individual's body is unique, and in this manner, every patient must work with a renal dietitian to think of an appropriately defined diet and well-crafted to the patient's needs.

The renal diet includes deteriorating and diminishing certain nutrients. A high sodium concentration can be destructive to individuals with kidney diseases because their kidneys can't enough dispose of an overabundance of sodium and liquid from the body. As sodium and fluid may rest and settle down in the tissues and circulatory system, it causes increased thirst, swollen legs, hands, face, high pulse, and heart disruptions and attacks. The abundance of liquid in the circulation system can exhaust your heart, making it augmented and feeble, and shortness of breath infers developing fluids in the lungs, making it hard to relax and breathe.

Maintain a crucial distance from table salt and high-sodium garnishes and toppings. Continuously attempt to cook at home, considering that most fast foods are high in sodium—attempt new flavors and herbs instead of salt to diminish and deal with your sodium intake. Attempt to avoid processed foods, if conceivable, because these bundled foods will, in general, be high in sodium. Always read the labels when shopping and picking foods that are low in sodium. Another route is to wash canned foods like veggies, beans, meats, and fish with water before serving.

If your kidneys cannot tackle potassium quantity, a patient must screen the measure of potassium that enters the body. Ask your primary care physician or dietitian if you have to restrict potassium. Your foods and drink decisions can assist you with bringing down your measures of potassium if necessary.

Salt substitutes can be high in potassium. Peruse the fixing mark. Check with your supplier about utilizing salt derivatives. Put a screening on canned foods before eating. More tips to help keep the degrees of potassium in your blood safe. Pick fresh foods grown from the ground and stay away from salt derivatives or subsidiaries and seasonings with potassium. Phosphorus can be found in numerous nourishments. Along these lines, patients with traded off kidney capacity should work with a renal dietitian to help oversee phosphorus levels.

It's a method for eating that shields your kidneys from further harm. It implies restricting a few ingredients and liquids to limit certain minerals by restrict their development in your body. Simultaneously, you'll need to ensure you get the right amount of protein, calories, nutrients, and minerals. In case you're in early periods of CKD, there might be scarcely any limits on what you can eat. But, as your infection deteriorates and dysfunction of kidneys prosper, you must be progressively cautious about what you consume or intake into your body.

CHAPTER 1

WHAT IS KIDNEY DISEASE

The kidneys maintain the fluids and water levels in the body. If you consume a lot of excess water, it is released out of the body by the kidneys. In the case of dehydration, more water is retained inside. All of this can happen if the kidneys are working properly. It can lead to toxic buildup in the body, damaging kidneys and other organs and disturbing the natural metabolism.

Most people are born with a kidney on each side of the body that simultaneously purifies the blood and supports each other in their renal function. Even when one kidney loses 40 percent of its renal function, the other kidney can hide this damage until properly checked and tested. This is why patients do not come to know about renal disease until there is enough damage done. If any of the kidneys lose its renal function below 25 percent, it must raise the alarms, which is highly dangerous. Individuals whose renal function decreases to only 15 percent would require an external treatment or dialysis.

Chronic kidney disease is a slow-moving disease and does not cause many complaints in the initial stages. The group of chronic kidney disease diseases includes several kidney diseases. The renal function decreases for several years or decades. With the help of timely diagnosis and treatment can slow down and even stop kidney disease progression.

In international studies of renal function in many people, it was found that almost every tenth kidney was found to have impaired kidney function to one degree or another.

COMMON CAUSES OF CHRONIC KIDNEY DISEASE

Diabetes - in the case of this disease, various organs are damaged, including the kidneys and heart and blood vessels, nerves, and eyes. With long-term diabetic kidney damage, many patients increase blood pressure and need to be treated accordingly.

High blood pressure (hypertension, primary arterial hypertension) - during hypertension, blood pressure cannot be controlled. It begins to exceed the limits of the norm (more than 140/90 mm Hg). If this condition is permanent, it can cause chronic kidney disease, brain stroke, or myocardial infarction.

Glomerulonephritis is a disease that occurs due to a breakdown in the immune system. The kidneys' filtration function disrupts immune inflammation. The disease can affect only the kidneys and spread to the entire body (vacuities, lupus nephritis). Glomerulonephritis is often accompanied by high blood pressure.

Many other conditions can cause chronic kidney disease, for example, hereditary diseases. Due to which many cysts appear in the kidneys, polycystic kidney disease damages renal tissue's functioning and develops renal failure. Other hereditary diseases of the kidneys are much fewer common problems caused by obstructions in the kidneys, and urine excretion - such as congenital malformations of the ureter, kidney stones, tumors, or enlargement of the prostate gland in men repeated urinary tract infections or pyelonephritis.

Does everyone have chronic kidney disease?

Chronic kidney disease can evolve at any age. The greatest risk of getting sick is in people who have one or more of the following risk factors:

- Diabetes
- High blood pressure
- Family members have kidney disease
- Age over 50
- Long-term consumption of drugs that can damage the kidneys
- Overweight or obesity

DIAGNOSE WITH CHRONIC KIDNEY DISEASE

There are two simple tests that your family doctor can prescribe to diagnose kidney disease.

BLOOD TEST:

Glomerular filtration rate (GFR) and serum creatinine level. Creatinine is one of those end products of protein metabolism. The blood level depends on age, gender, muscle mass, nutrition, physical activity, foods before taking the sample (for example, a lot of meat was eaten), and some drugs. Creatinine excretes from the body through the kidneys. Suppose the work of the kidneys slows down, the level of creatinine in the blood plasma increases.

Determining the creatinine level alone is insufficient for diagnosing chronic kidney disease since its value begins to exceed the upper limit of the norm only when GFR decreased by half. The creatinine reading, age, gender, and race of the patient. It shows at what level is the ability of the kidneys to filter. In chronic kidney disease, the GFR indicator indicates the stage of the severity of kidney disease.

URINE ANALYSIS:

The content of albumin in the urine is determined; also, albumin and creatinine values are determined by each other. Albumin is a protein in the urine that usually enters the urine in minimal quantities. Even a small increase in the level of albumin in the urine in some people may be an early sign of incipient kidney disease, especially in those with diabetes and high blood pressure. In normal kidney function, albumin in the urine should be no more than 3 mg/mmol (or 30 mg g). If albumin excretion increases even more, then it already speaks of kidney disease. If albumin excretion exceeds 300 mg g, other proteins are excreted into the urine, and this condition is called proteinuria.

If the kidney is healthy, then albumin does not enter the urine.

In the case of an injured kidney, albumin begins to enter the urine.

After receiving the urine analysis results, the doctor suspects that there is a kidney disease. An additional urine analysis is performed for albumin. If albuminuria or proteinuria is detected again within three months, it indicates chronic kidney disease.

ADDITIONAL EXAMINATIONS

In kidney ultrasound examination: in the diagnosis of chronic kidney disease, it is an examination of the primary choice. Ultrasound examination allows us to assess the kidneys' shape, size, location, and determine possible changes in the kidney tissue and other abnormalities that may interfere with the kidneys' normal functioning. Ultrasound examination of the kidneys does not require special training and has no risks for the patient.

If necessary, and if a urological disease is suspected, an ultrasound examination of the urinary tract can be prescribed (as well as a residual urine analysis). An ultrasound examination of the prostate gland can be prescribed for men and referred to a urologist for a consultation. If a gynecological disease is suspected, a woman is referred for consultation with a gynecologist.

You need to know about the examination with a contrast agent. If you have chronic kidney disease, diagnostic tests such as magnetic resonance imaging, computed tomography, and angiography are used to diagnose and treat various diseases and injuries. In many cases, intravenous and intra-arterial contrast agents (containing iodine or gadolinium) are used, making it possible to see the organs or blood vessels under study.

CHAPTER 2

HOW DOES KIDNEY WORK

The kidneys are found in the body's dorsal wall on the spine's sides. They are brown, weigh about 150 grams each, and are about 12 centimeters long, 6 centimeters wide, and 3 centimeters thick. In the upper part, each kidney has an endocrine gland attached (it produces vital substances inside the body) called the adrenal gland.

The kidneys are the cleaners where the blood is filtered and cleaned. They produce urine, which contains water, toxins, and salts that the blood has been collecting throughout the body, and that has to be eliminated. They also intervene in other activities such as reproduction because they have sex hormones; regulate the amount of phosphorus and calcium in the bones; they control the tension in the blood vessels, and manufacture substances involved in blood clotting.

Renal insufficiency appears when only 5 percent of the total kidney or nephron filters work. The kidney's basic unit is the nephron, of which there are about 1 million in each organ. Each nephron forms a component that acts as a filter, the glomerulus, and a transport system, the tubule.

Some of the blood that reaches the kidneys is filtered by the glomerulus and passes through the tubules. Various excretion and reabsorption processes occur that give rise to the urine that is eventually removed.

The renal blood flow (RBF or amount of blood reaching the kidney per minute) is approximately adult 1.1 liters per minute. The 0.6 liters plasma enter the glomerulus through the arterioles. The 20 percent is filtered, an operation called renal glomerular filtration.

Therefore, the renal glomerular filtrate is the volume of plasma filtered by the kidneys per unit of time. The amount of filtered plasma per day is 135 to 160 liters. To prevent fluid loss, between 98 percent and 99 percent of the renal glomerular filtration rate is reabsorbed by the tubules, resulting in the amount of urine removed from between one and two liters per day.

When a kidney disorder occurs, it means that one or more of the renal functions are altered. But not all functions are changed in the same proportion. If two-thirds of the nephrons cease to function, significant changes may not occur because the remaining nephrons adapt. Changes in hormonal production may go unnoticed. Then, renal glomerular filtration calculation is the only way to detect the decrease in the number of nephrons that continue to function.

Chronic renal failure or uremia is the kidneys' inability to produce urine or fabricate low quality ("like water") since it has not been removed enough toxic waste. Although some patients continue to urinate, most cannot. However, the important thing is not the quantity but the composition or quality of the urine.

Chronic kidney disease slowly worsens over time. In the early stages, it may be asymptomatic. Damage of function usually takes months to occur. When the person realizes, he is usually already with the functioning of the kidneys completely compromised.

Early symptoms of chronic renal failure usually also frequently occur in other diseases and may be the only signs of renal failure until it is advanced.

Symptoms may include:

- General malaise and fatigue
- Generalized itching (itching) and dry skin
- Headaches
- Unintentional Weight Loss
- Loss of appetite
- Nausea

Other symptoms that may appear, especially when kidney function worsens, include:

- Abnormally light or dark skin
- Bone pain
- Drowsiness and confusion
- Difficulty concentrating and reasoning
- Numbness in hands, feet, and other body areas
- Muscle spasms or cramps
- Bad breath
- Easy bruising, bleeding, or bloody stools
- Excessive thirst
- Frequent hiccups

- Low level of sexual interest and impotence
- Interruption of the menstrual period (amenorrhea)
- Sleep disorders
- Swelling of hands and legs (edema)
- Vomiting, usually in the morning

CHAPTER 3

UNDERSTANDING THE DIFFERENT TYPES OF KIDNEY FAILURE

K idney failure happens when your kidneys lose the capacity to channel waste from your blood adequately. Numerous variables can meddle with your kidney well-being and ability, such as dangerous presentation to natural toxins or certain drugs, certain intense and ceaseless infections, extreme drying out, and kidney injury. Your body gets over-burden with poisons if your kidneys can't do their standard employment. This can prompt kidney failure, which can be perilous whenever left untreated.

Somebody with kidney failure will possess a couple of symptoms of the disease. Once in a while, no symptoms are available. Potential symptoms incorporate a diminished measure of urination, swelling of your legs, lower legs, and feet from the maintenance of fluids brought about by the failure of the kidneys to wipe out water wastes, unexplained brevity of breath, over the top sleepiness or fatigue, steady sickness, confusion, and pain in your chest, seizures, and even outcome in extreme lethargies.

There are five types of kidney failure:

ACUTE PRE-RENAL KIDNEY FAILURE:

Deficient bloodstream to the kidneys can cause acute pre-renal kidney failure. The kidneys can't channel poisons from the blood without enough bloodstream. This sort of kidney failure can, as a rule, be restored once your primary care physician decides the reason for the diminished bloodstream.

ACUTE INTRINSIC KIDNEY FAILURE:

Acute inborn kidney failure can result from direct injury to the kidneys. Causes also incorporate poison, over-burden, and ischemia, a cut of oxygen supply to the kidneys. The ischemia might be the consequence of serious dying, stun, renal vein deterrent, and glomerulonephritis.

CHRONIC PRE-RENAL KIDNEY FAILURE:

When there isn't sufficient blood streaming to the kidneys for an all-encompassing timeframe, the kidneys start to fade and lose the capacity to work.

CHRONIC POST-RENAL KIDNEY FAILURE:

A long-haul blockage of the urinary tract averts urination. This causes pressure and inevitable kidney harm.

CHRONIC NATURAL KIDNEY FAILURE:

This happens when there's long haul harm to the kidneys because of characteristic kidney diseases. Natural kidney illness creates direct injury to the kidneys, for example, serious draining or absence of oxygen.

Different conditions can meddle with urine and potentially lead to kidney failure, including kidney stones, an expanded prostate, and blood clumps inside your urinary tract. It harms your nerves that control your bladder and some different things that may prompt kidney failure to incorporate blood or around your kidneys contamination.

If your kidneys are harmed or going towards harm at any spot, they may not function just as they should. If your kidneys' damage keeps on deteriorating and your kidneys are less ready to carry out their responsibility, you have chronic kidney diseases. Kidney failure is the last phase of an interminable kidney ailment. This is the reason kidney failure is likewise called end-stage renal disease, or ESRD for short.

SOME KIDNEY DISEASES

PYELONEPHRITIS:

Bacteria may contaminate the kidney. It can cause back pain and fever. A spread of microorganisms from untreated bladder contamination is the most widely recognized reason for pyelonephritis.

KIDNEY STONES (NEPHROLITHIASIS):

It is minerals in urine structure some crystals, which may develop sufficiently enormous to block urine passageway. It's viewed as one of the most deteriorating conditions. Most kidney stones pass alone. However, some are excessively huge and should be dealt with.

GLOMERULONEPHRITIS:

An overactive resistant framework may assault the kidney, causing aggravation and a little harm. Blood and protein in the urine are basic issues that happen with glomerulonephritis. It can likewise extend up to kidney failure.

NEPHROTIC DISORDER:

Damage to the kidneys makes them spill a lot of protein into the urine. Edema might be a symptom of this disease.

POLYCYSTIC KIDNEY MALADY:

A hereditary condition bringing about huge sores in the two kidneys that obstruct their functioning.

ACUTE RENAL FAILURE:

An unexpected decline in how well your kidneys work. Lack of hydration, a blockage in the urinary tract, or kidney harm can cause acute renal failure, which might or might not be reversed.

CHRONIC RENAL FAILURE:

A long-lasting fractional loss of how well your kidneys work. The most widely recognized causes are diabetes and hypertension.

END-STAGE RENAL DISEASE (ESRD):

Complete loss of kidney functioning and proper structure, as a rule, because of dynamic chronic kidney disorder. Individuals with ESRD require standard dialysis for endurance.

PAPILLARY NECROSIS:

Severe harm to the kidneys can cause lumps of kidney tissue to sever inside and obstruct the kidneys. If that goes untreated, the subsequent damage can prompt all-out kidney failure.

DIABETIC NEPHROPATHY:

High glucose from diabetes logically harms the kidneys, in the end, causing interminable kidney diseases. Protein in the urine may likewise result in this disease to happen.

HYPERTENSIVE NEPHROPATHY:

Kidney harm brought about by hypertension. Chronic renal failure may be the result.

KIDNEY CANCER:

Renal cell carcinoma is the most widely recognized disease influencing the kidney. Smoking is the most well-known reason for kidney cancer.

INTERSTITIAL NEPHRITIS:

Infections of the connective tissue inside the kidney, frequently causing acute renal failure. Unfavorably susceptible responses and medication reactions are common causes.

MINIMAL CHANGE DISEASE:

A type of Nephrotic disorder in which kidney cells look practically normal under the magnifying lens or microscope. The condition can cause significant leg swelling. Steroids are utilized to treat these minimal change diseases.

NEPHROGENIC DIABETES INSIPIDUS:

The kidneys lose the capacity to formulate the urine, as a consequence, because of some drug habits or irregularities. Although it's once in a while risky, diabetes insipidus causes thirst and frequent urination.

RENAL CYST:

Separated kidney cysts regularly occur as an individual's age grows, and they never cause an issue. Complex growths and masses can be destructive.

CHAPTER 4

UNDERSTANDING IF YOUR KIDNEYS HAVE FAILED

A kidney disease diagnosis can seem devastating at first. The news may come as a shock for some people who may not have experienced any symptoms. It's important to remember that you can control your progress and improvement through diet and lifestyle changes, even when a prognosis is serious. Taking steps to improve your health can make a significant effort to slow kidney disease progression and improve your life quality.

FOCUS ON WEIGHT LOSS

Losing weight is one of the most common reasons for going on a diet. It's also one of the best ways to treat kidney disease and prevent further damage. Carrying excess weight contributes to high toxicity levels in the body by storing toxins instead of releasing them through the kidneys. Eating foods high in trans fats, sugar, and excess sodium contributes to obesity, affecting close to one-third of North Americans and continues to rise in many other countries, where fast foods are becoming easier to access and less expensive. Losing weight is a difficult cycle for many, who often diet temporarily only to return to unhealthy habits after reaching a milestone, which results in gaining the weight back, thus causing a harmful yo-yo diet effect.

There are some necessary and easy changes you can make to shed those first pounds, which will begin to take the pressure off the kidneys and help you onto the path of regular weight loss:

- Drink plenty of water. If you can't drink eight glasses a day, try adding unsweetened natural sparkling water or herbal teas to increase your water intake.

- Limit the sugar and carbohydrates you consume. This doesn't require adapting to a ketogenic or low-carb diet – you'll notice a significant change after ditching soda and reducing the bread and pasta by half.
- Take your time to eat and avoid rushing. If you need to eat in a hurry, grab a piece of fruit or a small portion of macadamia nuts. Avoid sugary and salty foods as much as possible. Choose fresh fruits over potato chips and chocolate bars.
- Create a shortlist of kidney-friendly foods that you enjoy and use this as your reference or guide when grocery shopping. This will help you stock up on snacks, ingredients, and foods for your kitchen that work well within your renal diet plan, at the same time reducing your chances of succumbing to the temptation of eating a bag of salted pretzels or chocolate.

Once you make take a few steps towards changing the way you eat, it will get easier. Making small changes at first is the key to success and progress with a new eating and living way. If you are already in the habit of consuming packaged foods – such as crackers, chips, processed dips, sauces, and sodas, for example – try cutting down on one or two items at a time, and over some time, gradually eliminate and cut down other items. Slowly replace these with fresh foods and healthier choices so that your body has a chance to adapt without extreme cravings that often occur during sudden changes.

QUIT SMOKING AND REDUCE ALCOHOL

It's not easy to quit smoking or using recreational drugs, especially where there has been long-term use and the effects have already impacted your health. At some point, you'll begin to notice a difference in the way you feel and how your body changes over time. This includes chronic coughing related to respiratory conditions, shortness of breath, and a lack of energy. Smoking inevitably catches up with age and contributes to cancer, premature aging, and kidney damage. The more toxins we consume or add to our body, the more challenging it becomes for the kidneys to work efficiently, which eventually slows their ability to function.

For most people, quitting "cold turkey" or all at once is not an option because of the withdrawal symptoms and increased chances of starting again. However, this method can work if applied with a strong support system and a lot of determination, though it's not the best option for everyone. Reducing smoking on your own, or switching to e-cigarettes or a patch or medication, can help significantly over time. Setting goals of reduction until the point of quitting can be a beneficial way to visualize success and provide a sense of motivation. The following tips may also be useful for quitting smoking and other habit-forming substances:

- Join a support group and talk to other people who relate to you. Share your struggles, ideas, and thoughts, which will help others and yourself during this process.

- Track your progress on a calendar or in a notebook, either by pen and paper, or on an application. This can serve as a motivator to display how you've done so far and where you can improve. For example, you may have reduced your smoking from ten to seven cigarettes per day, then increased to nine. This may indicate a slight change that can keep in mind to focus on reducing your intake further, from nine cigarettes to seven or six per day, and so on.
- Be aware of stressors in your life that cause you to smoke or use substances. If these factors are avoidable, make every effort to minimize or stop them from impacting your life. This may include specific people, places, or situations that can "trigger" a craving or make you feel more likely to use than usual. If there are situations that you cannot avoid, such as family, work, or school-related problems, consult with a trusted friend or someone you can confide in who can be present with you during these instances.
- Don't be afraid to ask for help. Many people cannot quit on their own without at least some assistance from others. Seeking a counselor or medical professional's guidance and expertise to better yourself can be one of the most important decisions you make to improve the quality of your life.

GETTING ACTIVE

Staying active and regular exercise is essential ways to keep fit and healthy. Regular movement is critical, and training is different for everyone, depending on their abilities and options. Fortunately, there are unlimited ways to customize an exercise routine or plan that can suit any lifestyle, perhaps low impact to start, or if you're ready, engage in a more vigorous workout. For many people experiencing kidney disease, one of the significant struggles is losing weight and living a sedentary life.

The movement is generally minimal, and exercise is usually not commonly practiced. Smoking, eating processed foods, and not getting the required nutrition can further impair the body so that exercise is seen as a hurdle and a challenge that is best avoided. Making lifestyle changes is not something that should be done all at once, but over some time – especially during the early stages of renal disease – so that the condition's impact is minimized over time and becomes more manageable.

Where can you begin if you haven't exercised at all or for an extended period? For starters, don't sign up for a marathon or engage in any strenuous activities unless it is safe to do so. Start slow and take your time. Before taking on any new movements, always talk to your doctor to rule out any impact this may have on other existing conditions, such as blood pressure and respiratory diseases, as well as your kidneys. Most, if not all, physicians will likely recommend exercise as part of the treatment plan but may advise beginning slowly if your body isn't used to exercise.

Simple techniques to introduce exercise into your life require a commitment. This can begin with a quick 15-minute walk or jog and a 10-or 15-minute stretch in the morning before starting your day. There are some easy, introductory techniques to consider, including the following:

- Take a walk for 10 to 15 minutes each day, at least three or four days each week. If you find it difficult at first, due to cramping, respiratory issues, or other conditions, walk slowly and breathe deeply. Make sure you feel relaxed during your walks. Find a scenic path or area in your neighborhood that is pleasant and gives you something to enjoy, such as a beautiful sunset or forested park.
- Stretch for five minutes once a day. This doesn't mean you need to do any intricate yoga poses or specific techniques. Moving your ankles, wrists, and arms in circles and standing every so often (if you sit often), and twisting your torso can help release stress, improve your blood flow, lower blood pressure, and help your body transport nutrients areas in need of repair.
- Practice breathing long, measured breaths. This will help prepare you for more endurance-based exercise, such as jogging, long walks, cycling, and swimming. Count to five on each inhale and exhale. Practice moving as you breathe, sync, or coordinate your body's movements with your breathing. If you have difficulty with the respiratory system, take it slow and don't push yourself. If you feel weak or out of breath, stop immediately and try again later or the following day at a slower pace.
- Start a beginner's yoga class and learn the fundamentals of various poses and stretches. It is helpful to arrive early and speak with the instructor, who can provide guidance on which modifications work best if needed. They can also give tips on approaching certain poses or movements that can be challenging for beginners so that you feel more comfortable and knowledgeable before you start.
- If you smoke, exercise will present more of a challenge on your lungs and respiratory function. Once you become accustomed to a beginner's level and become moderately active, you may notice it takes more effort, which requires an increase in lung capacity and oxygen. Smoking will eventually present a challenge. Where quitting can be a long-term and challenging goal in itself, please make an effort to cut back as much as it takes to allow your body's movements and exercise to continue.

Once you get into a basic routine, there is a wide variety of individual and team activities to consider for your life. Joining a baseball team or badminton club may be ideal. For more solitary options, consider swimming, cycling, or jogging. Many gyms and community centers provide monthly plans and may offer a free trial period to see if their facilities work for you. This is an excellent opportunity to try new classes and equipment to gauge how much you can achieve, even if in the early stages of exercise, so that you can decide whether to pursue dance aerobics, spin classes, and weight training. Some gyms will provide a free consultation with a personal trainer to set a simple plan towards weight loss and strength training goals.

CHAPTER 5

RENAL DIET AND IT BENEFITS

ietary control, including protein, phosphorus, and sodium limitation, can impact perpetual renal patients by following conventional and nontraditional cardiovascular hazard factors.

Circulatory strain control might be supported by the decrease of sodium consumption and the vegan idea of the eating routine, which is significant for bringing down serum cholesterol and improving the plasma lipid profile.

Protein-limited eating regimens may have likewise calming and against oxidant properties.

The general principles of diet treatment for chronic kidney patients are as follows:

- Limit protein intake to 0.8 gm/kg per kilogram per day for non-dialysis patients. Patients on dialysis need a greater amount of protein to compensate for the possible loss of proteins during the procedure. (1.0 to 1.2 gm/kg daily according to body weight)
- Take enough carbohydrates to provide energy
- Take average amounts of oil—reduction of butter, pure fat, and oil intake.
- Restriction of fluid and water intake in case of swelling (edema)
- Dietary intake of sodium, potassium, and phosphorus limitation
- Take adequate amounts of vitamins and trace elements. A high-fiber diet is recommended.

The details of the selection and modification of the diet for chronic kidney patients are as follows:

HIGH-CALORIE INTAKE

In addition to daily activities to maintain heat, growth, and body weight the body needs calories. Calories are taken with carbohydrates and fats. According to body weight, the daily average calorie intake of patients suffering from chronic kidney disease is 35-40 kcal/kg. If caloric intake is insufficient, the body uses proteins to provide calories. Such protein distribution may cause harmful effects, such as improper nutrition and increased production of waste materials. Therefore, it is essential to provide sufficient calories to CKD patients. It is essential to calculate the patient's daily calorie requirement based on the ideal body weight, not the current value.

CARBOHYDRATES

Carbohydrates are the primary source of calories required for the body. Diabetes and obesity patients should limit the number of carbohydrates. It is best to use complex carbohydrates that can be obtained from whole grains such as whole wheat or raw rice that can provide fiber. They should constitute a large part of the number of carbohydrates in the diet. The proportion of all other sugar-containing substances should not exceed 20% of the total carbohydrate intake, particularly in diabetic patients. As long as chocolate, hazelnut, or banana desserts are consumed in a limited amount, non-diabetic patients may be replaced with calories, fruit, pies, pastry, cookies, and protein.

OILS

Fats are a source of calories for the body and provide twice as many carbohydrates and proteins. Chronic kidney patients should limit the intake of saturated fat and cholesterol that may cause heart disease. In unsaturated fat, it is necessary to pay attention to the proportion of monounsaturated fat and polyunsaturated fat. Excessive uptake of omega-6 polyunsaturated fatty acids (CFAs) and a relatively high omega-6 / omega-3 ratio are detrimental, while the low omega-6 / omega-3 ratio has beneficial effects. The use of vegetable oils instead of uniform oils will achieve this goal. Trans fat-containing substances such as potato chips, sweet buns, instant cookies, and pastries are extremely dangerous and should be avoided.

RESTRICTION OF PROTEIN INTAKE

Protein is essential for the restoration and maintenance of body tissues. It also helps to heal wounds and fight infection. In patients with chronic renal failure who do not undergo dialysis, protein limitation is recommended to reduce the rate of decrease in renal function and postpone the need for dialysis and renal transplantation. (<0.8 gm/kg daily according to body weight). However, excessive protein restriction should also be avoided due to the risk of malnutrition.

Anorexia is a common condition in patients with chronic kidney disease. Strict protein restriction, low diet, weight loss, fatigue, loss of body resistance, and loss of appetite increase the risk of death. High proteins such as meat, poultry, and fish, eggs, and tofu are preferred. Chronic kidney patients should avoid high protein diets. Similarly, protein supplements or medications such as creatinine used for muscle development should be avoided unless recommended by a physician or dietician. However, as the patient begins dialysis, daily protein intake should be increased by 1.0 to 1.2 gm/kg body weight to recover the proteins lost during the procedure.

FLUID INTAKE

Why should chronic kidney patients take precautions about fluid intake?

The kidneys are essential in maintaining the correct amount of water in the body by removing excess liquid as urea. In patients with chronic kidney disease, the urea volume usually decreases as the kidney functions deteriorate. Reduction of urea excretion from the body causes fluid retention in the body, resulting in facial swelling, swelling of legs and hands, and high blood pressure. A build-up of fluid in the lungs causes shortness of breath and difficulty breathing. It can be life-threatening if not checked.

What precautions should chronic kidney patients take to control fluid intake?

The amount of fluid taken on a physician's advice should be recorded and monitored to prevent overloading or loss of fluid. The amount of water to be taken for each chronic kidney patient may vary, and this rate is calculated according to the urea excretion and fluid status of each patient.

What is the recommended amount of fluid for patients with chronic kidney disease?

Unlimited edema and water intake can be done in patients who do not have edema and can throw enough urea from the body. It is a common misconception that patients with kidney disease should take large amounts of water and fluids to protect their kidneys. The recommended amount of liquid depends on the patient's clinical condition and renal function.

Patients with edema who cannot appoint sufficient urea from the body should limit fluid intake. To reduce swelling, fluid intake within 24 hours should be less than the amount of urine produced by the daily body.

In patients with edema, the amount of fluid that should be taken daily should be 500 ml more than the previous day's urine volume to prevent fluid overload or fluid loss. This additional 500 ml of liquid will approximately compensate for the fluids lost by perspiration and exhalation.

Why should chronic kidney patients keep a record of their daily weight?

Patients need to record their weight daily to detect fluid increase or loss or to monitor fluid volume in their bodies. Bodyweight will remain constant if the instructions for fluid intake are strictly followed. Sudden weight gain indicates excessive fluid overload due to increased fluid intake in the body. Weight gain is a warning that the patient should make more rigorous fluid restriction. Weight loss is usually caused by fluid restriction and the use of diuretics.

USEFUL TIPS FOR RESTRICTING FLUID INTAKE

Reduce salty, spicy, or fried foods in your diet because these foods can increase your thirst and cause more fluid consumption.

Only for water when you are thirsty. Do not drink as a habit or because everyone drinks.

When thirsty, consume only a small amount of water or try ice — sure, taking a little ice cube. Ice stays in the mouth longer than water to give a more satisfying result than the same amount of water. Remember to calculate the amount of liquid consumed. To calculate, freeze the amount of water allocated for drinking in the ice block.

To prevent dry mouth, gargle with water, but do not swallow the water. Dry mouth can also be reduced by chewing gum, sucking hard candies, lemon slices, or mint candies, and using a small amount of water to moisturize your mouth.

Always use small cups or glasses to limit fluid intake. Instead of consuming extra water for medication use, take your medicines while drinking water after meals.

High blood sugar in diabetic patients can increase the level of thirst. It is essential to keep blood sugar under tight control to reduce hunger.

Since the person's thirst increases in hot weather, measures to be in more relaxed environments may be preferred and recommended.

CHAPTER 6

KIDNEY FAILURE TREATMENT

The physician will decide whether you belong to any of the high-risk groups. They're going to run some tests to see if your kidneys are working properly. The following tests may include:

Glomerular filtration rate (GFR) - This test will assess how well the kidneys are functioning and kidney disease level or kidney failure.

Ultrasound or computed tomography (CT) Ultrasound and CT scans will show clear images of your kidneys and urinary tract.

KIDNEY BIOPSY

Your health care provider can remove a piece of tissue from your kidney during a kidney biopsy while you're sleeping. The tissue sample will help the healthcare provider understand what type of kidney disease you have and how much damage has occurred.

URINE TEST

Your doctor may request a sample of urine for albumin testing. Albumin is a protein that can be transmitted to your urine when it damages your kidneys.

BLOOD CREATININE TEST

Creatinine is a product of waste. Once creatine (a protein in the muscle) is broken down, it will be released into the blood. If your kidneys don't work properly, the creatinine levels in your blood will increase.

With chronic kidney disease, there is no current or permanent treatment. However, some treatment methods or medication can aid control signs and symptoms, delay disease progression, and reduce complications.

Patients suffering from chronic kidney disease need to take a significant number of medications.

TREATMENTS

ANEMIA TREATMENT

Hemoglobin is the material that comes with essential oxygen around the body in red blood cells. If there are low levels of hemoglobin, the patient will have anemia.

Most kidney anemia patients may need blood transfusion. In general, iron supplements must be taken by a person suffering from kidney disease, whether via routine ferrous sulfate tablets or injections.

PHOSPHATE BALANCE

Persons with kidney disease may not be able to extract phosphate from their bodies properly. Patients are guided to decrease their nutritional phosphate intake, like dairy products, red meat, eggs, and fish consumption.

HYPERTENSION

High blood pressure is a widespread problem for patients with chronic kidney failure. It is important to reduce blood pressure to protect the kidneys and then slow down the disease's progression.

SHORTENING SKIN

Antihistamines, such as chlorphenamine, can help relieve itching symptoms.

MEDICINES AGAINST THE DISEASE

If toxins accumulate in the body because the kidneys are not functioning correctly, patients may feel sick (nausea). Medications such as cyclin or metoclopramide help relieve the disease.

NSAIDS (NON-STEROIDAL ANTI-INFLAMMATORY DRUGS)

NSAIDs, including aspirin or ibuprofen, should be avoided and taken only if a doctor recommends them.

TERMINAL TREATMENT

This is when the kidneys function at less than 10% to 15% of their standard capacity. Measures used to date (diet, medication, and treatments that control the underlying issues) will no longer be available. The kidneys of patients with end-stage renal failure cannot cope with the process of waste and fluid removal: the patient will need dialysis or a kidney transplant to survive.

Most doctors will try to delay dialysis or kidney transplant as much as possible since they carry the risk of potentially serious complications.

RENAL DIALYSIS

A peritoneal dialysis is a treatment option for chronic kidney disease.

There are two main types of renal dialysis. Each class also has subtypes. The two main types are:

Hemodialysis: The blood is pumped from the patient's body and passes through dialysis (an artificial kidney). The patient undergoes hemodialysis approximately three times a week. Each session lasts a minimum of 3 hours.

Experts now identify that more frequent sessions result in a better quality of life for the patient, but modern home dialysis techniques make the regular use of hemodialysis possible.

Peritoneal dialysis: Blood enters the patient's abdomen; in the peritoneal cavity containing an extensive network of small blood vessels. A catheter is implanted in the stomach. The dialysis solution is infused and drained for as long as necessary to eliminate waste and excess fluid.

KIDNEY TRANSPLANT

The kidney donor and recipient must have the same blood type, cell surface proteins, and antibodies to reduce the risk of rejection of the new kidney. The best types of donors are typical brothers or close relatives. When it is impossible to have a living donor, the search for a dead donor must begin.

DRUGS AND MEDICINES

Your doctor will prescribe angiotensin-converting enzymes (ACE) inhibitors, such as lisinopril and ramipril. Or angiotensin receptor blockers (BRA), such as irbesartan and Olmesartan. These are blood pressure drugs that can slow down the progression of kidney disease. Your doctor may prescribe these medications to help you maintain your kidney function, even if you do not have high blood pressure.

It can also be treated with cholesterol medications (such as simvastatin). These medications can bring down blood cholesterol levels and help to maintain your kidney health properly. Depending on your symptoms observed, your doctor may also prescribe medication to relieve inflammation and treat anemia.

CHAPTER 7

LEARNING TO DEAL WITH KIDNEY FAILURE

During kidney disease, this is extremely important. They can advise you about sodium, phosphorous, and potassium content of favorite foods and recommend reducing your sodium intake. Your diet will be tailored to you, considering the stage of kidney disease you're in and any other illnesses or diseases you suffer from.

KEEP A FOOD DIARY

You should track what you're eating and drinking to stay within the guidelines and recommendations given to you. Apps such as My Fitness Pal make this extremely easy and even track many of the minerals and levels in foods, including sodium, protein, etc. There are also apps specifically made for kidney disease patients to track sodium, phosphorous, and potassium levels.

READ FOOD LABELS

Some foods have hidden sodium in them, even if they don't taste salty. You will need to cut back on the amount of canned, frozen, and processed foods you eat. Check your beverages for added sodium.

CHECK FOOD LABELS TO AVOID

Potassium chloride, Tetrasodium phosphate, Sodium phosphate, Trisodium phosphate, Tricalcium phosphate, Phosphoric acid, Polyphosphate, Hexametaphosphate, Pyrophosphate, Monocalcium phosphate, Dicalcium phosphate, Aluminum phosphate, Sodium tripolyphosphate, Sodium polyphosphate.

FLAVOR FOODS WITH SPICES AND HERBS RATHER THAN SHOP-BOUGHT DRESSINGS AND CONDIMENTS

These add flavor and variety to your meals and are not packed with sodium; spices also have many health benefits. Stay away from salt substitutes and seasonings that contain potassium. Use citrus fruits and vinegar for dressings and to add flavor.

KEEP UP YOUR APPOINTMENTS WITH YOUR DOCTOR OR NEPHROLOGIST

Let your doctor know if you notice any swelling or changes in your weight.

MONITOR DRINK AND FLUID INTAKE

You have probably been told you need to drink up to eight glasses of water a day. This is true for a healthy body, but for people experiencing the later stages of CKD, these fluids can build up and cause additional problems. The restriction of fluids will differ from person to person. Things to take into consideration are swelling urine output and weight gain. Your weight will be recorded before dialysis begins, and once it's over. This is done to determine how much fluid to remove from your body. If you are undergoing hemodialysis, this will be recorded approximately three times a week. If you are undergoing peritoneal dialysis, your weight is recorded every day. If there is a significant weight gain, you may be drinking too many fluids.

MEASURE PORTION SIZES

Moderating your portion sizes is essential. Use smaller cups, bowls, or plates to avoid giving yourself oversized portions.

Measure your food so you can keep an accurate record of how much you are eating:

- The size of a fist is equal to 1 cup.
- The palm is equal to 3 ounces.
- The tip of your thumb is equivalent to 1 teaspoon.
- A poker chip is equal to 1 tablespoon.

Substitution Tips:

- Use plain white flour instead of whole-wheat/whole-grain
- Use all-purpose flour instead of self-raising,
- Use Stevia instead of sugar,

- Use egg whites rather than whole eggs,
- Use soy milk or almond rice instead of cow's milk.

OTHER ADVICE

Be careful when eating in restaurants -ask for dressings and condiments on the side and watch out for soups and cured meats.

- Watch out for convenience foods that are high in sodium.
- Prepare your meals and freeze them for future use.
- Drain liquids from canned vegetables and fruits to help control potassium levels.

CHAPTER 8

FOODS TO EAT
AND TO AVOID

FOOD TO EAT

The renal diet aims to cut down the amount of waste in the blood. When people have kidney dysfunction, the kidneys are unable to remove and filter waste properly. When waste is left in the blood, it can affect the electrolyte levels of the patient. With a kidney diet, kidney function is promoted, and the progression of complete kidney failure is slowed down.

The renal diet follows a low intake of protein, phosphorus, and sodium. It is necessary to consume high-quality protein and limit some fluids. For some people, it is important to limit calcium and potassium.

Promoting a renal diet, here are the substances which are critical to be monitored:

SODIUM AND ITS ROLE IN THE BODY

Most natural foods contain sodium. Some people think that sodium and salt are interchangeable. However, salt is a compound of chloride and sodium. There might be either salt or sodium in other forms in the food we eat. Due to the added salt, processed foods include a higher level of sodium.

Apart from potassium and chloride, sodium is one of the most crucial body's electrolytes. The main function of electrolytes is to control the fluids when they are going out and in the body's cells and tissues.

With sodium:

- Blood volume and pressure are regulated.
- Muscle contraction and nerve function are regulated.

- The acid-base balance of the blood is regulated.
- The amount of fluid the body eliminates and keeps is balanced.

Why is it important to monitor sodium intake for people with kidney issues?

Since the kidneys of kidney disease patients are unable to reduce excess fluid and sodium from the body adequately, too much sodium might be harmful. As fluid and sodium build up in the bloodstream and tissues, they might cause:

- Edema: swelling in face, hands, and legs
- Increased thirst
- High blood pressure
- Shortness of breath
- Heart failure

The ways to monitor sodium intake:

- Avoid processed foods
- Be attentive to serving sizes.
- Read food labels
- Utilize fresh meats instead of processed
- Choose fresh fruits and veggies.
- Compare brands, choosing the ones with the lowest sodium levels.
- Utilize spices that do not include salt
- Ensure the sodium content is less than 400 mg per meal and not more than 150 mg per snack
- Cook at home, not adding salt
- Foods to eat with lower sodium content:
- Fresh meats, dairy products, frozen veggies, and fruits
- Fresh herbs and seasonings like rosemary, oregano, dill, lime, cilantro, onion, lemon, and garlic
- Corn tortilla chips, pretzels, no salt added crackers, unsalted popcorn

POTASSIUM AND ITS ROLE IN THE BODY

The main function of potassium is keeping muscles working correctly and the heartbeat regular. This mineral is responsible for maintaining electrolyte and fluid balance in the bloodstream. The kidneys regulate the proper amount of potassium in the body, expelling excess amounts in the urine.

Monitoring potassium intake

- Limit high potassium food

- Select only fresh fruits and veggies
- Limit dairy products and milk to 8 oz per day
- Avoid potassium chloride
- Read labels on packaged foods.
- Avoid seasonings and salt substitutes with potassium.

Foods to eat with lower potassium:

- Fruits: watermelon, tangerines, pineapple, plums, peaches, pears, papayas, mangoes, lemons and limes, honeydew, grapefruit/grapefruit juice, grapes/grape juice, clementine/satsuma, cranberry juice, berries, and apples/ applesauce, apple juice
- Veggies: summer squash (cooked), okra, mushrooms (fresh), lettuce, kale, green beans, eggplant, cucumber, corn, onions (raw), celery, cauliflower, carrots, cabbage, broccoli (fresh), bamboo shoots (canned), and bell peppers
- Plain Turkish delights, marshmallows and jellies, boiled fruit sweets, and peppermints
- Shortbread, ginger nut biscuits, plain digestives
- Plain flapjacks and cereal bars
- Plain sponge cakes like Madeira cake, lemon sponge, jam sponge
- Corn-based and wheat crisps
- Whole grain crispbreads and crackers
- Protein and other foods (bread (not whole grain), pasta, noodles, rice, eggs, canned tuna, turkey (white meat), and chicken (white meat)

PHOSPHORUS AND ITS ROLE IN THE BODY

This mineral is essential in bone development and maintenance. Phosphorus helps in the development of connective organs and tissue and assists in muscle movement. Extra phosphorus is possible to be removed by healthy kidneys. However, it is impossible with kidney dysfunction. High levels of phosphorus make bones weak by pulling calcium out of your bones. It might lead to dangerous calcium deposits in the heart, eyes, lungs, and blood vessels.

Monitoring phosphorus intake

- Pay attention to serving size
- Eat fresh fruits and veggies
- Eat smaller portions of foods that are rich in protein
- Avoid packaged foods
- Keep a food journal

Foods to eat with low phosphorus level:

- grapes, apples
- lettuce, leeks
- Carbohydrates (white rice, corn, and rice Cereal, popcorn, pasta, crackers (not wheat), white bread)
- Meat (sausage, fresh meat)

PROTEIN

Damaged kidneys are unable to remove protein waste, so they accumulate in the blood. The amount of protein to consume differs depending on the stage of CKD. Protein is critical for tissue maintenance, and it is necessary to eat the proper amount of it according to the particular stage of kidneys disease.

Sources of protein for vegetarians:

- Vegans (allowing only plant-based foods): Wheat protein and whole grains, nut butter, soy protein, yogurt or soy milk, cooked no salt added canned and dried beans and peas, unsalted nuts.
- Lacto vegetarians (allowing dairy products, milk, and plant-based foods): reduced-sodium or low-sodium cottage cheese.
- Lacto-Ovo vegetarians (allowing eggs, dairy products, milk, and plant-based foods): eggs.

FOOD TO AVOID

Food with high sodium content:

- Onion salt, marinades, garlic salt, teriyaki sauce, and table salt
- Pepperoni, bacon, ham, lunch meat, hot dogs, sausage, processed meats
- Ramen noodles, canned produce, and canned soups
- Marinara sauce, gravy, salad dressings, soy sauce, BBQ sauce, and ketchup
- Chex Mix, salted nuts, Cheetos, crackers, and potato chips
- Fast food

Food with a high potassium level:

- Fruits: dried fruit, oranges/orange juice, prunes/prune juice, kiwi, nectarines, dates, cantaloupe, bananas, black currants, damsons, cherries, grapes, and apricots.
- Vegetables: tomatoes/tomato sauce/tomato juice, sweet potatoes, beans, lentils, split peas, spinach (cooked), pumpkin, potatoes, mushrooms (cooked), chile peppers, chard, Brussels sprouts (cooked), broccoli (cooked), baked beans, avocado, butternut squash, and acorn squash.

- Protein and other foods: peanut butter, molasses, granola, chocolate, bran, sardines, fish, bacon, ham, nuts and seeds, yogurt, milkshakes, and milk.
- Coconut-based snacks, nut-based snacks, fudge, and toffee
- Cakes containing marzipan.
- Potato crisps.

Foods with high phosphorus:

- Dairy products: pudding, ice cream, yogurt, cottage cheese, cheese, and milk
- Nuts and seeds: sunflower seeds, pumpkin seeds, pecans, peanut butter, pistachios, cashews, and almonds
- Dried beans and peas: soybeans, split peas, refried beans, pinto beans, lentils, kidney beans, garbanzo beans, black beans, and baked beans.
- Meat: veal, turkey, liver, lamb, beef, bacon, fish, and seafood.
- Carbohydrates: whole grain products, oatmeal, and bran cereals

RENAL DIET SHOPPING LIST

VEGETABLES:

- Arugula (raw)
- Alfalfa sprouts
- Bamboo shoots
- Asparagus
- Beans - pinto, wax, fava, green
- Bean sprouts
- Bitter melon (balsam pear)
- Beet greens (raw)
- Broccoli
- Broad beans (boiled, fresh)
- Cactus
- Cabbage - red, swamp, Napa/ Suey Choy, skunk
- Carrots
- Calabash
- Celery
- Cauliflower
- Chayote
- Celeriac (cooked)
- Collard greens
- Chicory
- Cucumber
- Corn
- Okra
- Onions
- Pepitas
- (Green) Peas
- Peppers
- Radish
- Radicchio
- Seaweed
- Rapini (raw)
- Shallots
- Spinach (raw)
- Snow peas
- Dandelion greens (raw)
- Daikon
- Plant Leaves
- Drumstick
- Endive

- Eggplant
- Fennel bulb
- Escarole
- Fiddlehead greens
- Ferns
- Hearts of Palm
- Irish moss
- Hominy
- Jicama, raw
- Leeks
- Kale(raw)
- Mushrooms (raw white)
- Lettuce (raw)

- Mustard greens
- Swiss chard (raw)
- Squash
- Turnip
- Tomatillos (raw)
- Watercress
- Turnip greens
- Wax beans
- Water chestnuts (canned)
- Winter melon
- Wax gourd
- Zucchini (raw)

FRUITS:

- Acerola Cherries
- Apple
- Blackberries
- Asian Pear
- Boysenberries
- Blueberries
- Cherries
- Casaba melon
- Clementine
- Chokeberries
- Crabapples
- Cloudberries
- Cranberries (fresh)
- Grapefruit
- Gooseberries
- Pomegranate
- Grapes
- Rambutan
- Quince
- Rhubarb
- Raspberries (fresh or frozen)
- Jujubes
- Golden Berry

- Kumquat
- Jackfruit
- Lingonberries
- Lemon
- Loganberries
- Lime
- Lychees
- Mango
- Mandarin orange
- Peach
- Pineapple
- Pear
- Plum
- Strawberries
- Rose-apple
- Tangerine
- Tangelo
- Watermelon

FRESH MEAT, SEAFOOD, AND POULTRY:

- Chicken
- Beef and Ground Beef
- Goat
- Duck
- Wild Game

- Pork
- Lamb
- Veal
- Turkey
- Fish

MILK, EGGS, AND DAIRY:

Milk:

- Milk (½-1 cup/day)

Non-Dairy Milk:

- Almond Fresh (Original, Unsweetened, Vanilla)
- Almond Breeze (Original, Vanilla, Vanilla Unsweetened, Original Unsweetened)
- Silk True Almond Beverage (Unsweetened Original, Original, Vanilla, Unsweetened Vanilla)
- Good Karma Flax Delight (Vanilla, Original, Unsweetened)
- Rice Dream Rice Drink (Vanilla Classic, Non-Enriched Original Classic)
- Silk Soy Beverage (Original, Vanilla, Unsweetened)
- Natura Organic Fortified Rice Beverage (Original, Vanilla)
- PC Organics Fortified Rice Beverage

Other Dairy Products:

- Non-Hydrogenated Margarine (Salt-Free or Regular)
- Butter (Unsalted or Regular)
- Whipping Cream
- Sour Cream
- Whipped Cream

CHAPTER 9

JUICE AND BEVERAGES FOR THE RENAL DIET

FRESH JUICES

There are plenty of delicious, thirst-quenching drinks available on the renal diet. It includes various teas and juices, both vegetable and fruit-based, to ensure you get the nutrients you need while helping your kidneys with the detoxification process. When choosing a juice, ensure that it's as natural as possible and freshly squeezed or pressed, if this option is available. Juices and smoothies can be squeezed, or prepared in a blender, though a freshly pressed juice is a best and easiest option.

POMEGRANATE JUICE

A tangy, delicious fruit, pomegranate is an excellent source of vitamin C and fiber. It's a great tasting snack on its own, sliced into quarters. The seeds have a variety of nutrients, including antioxidants. Juicing pomegranate is easily done with an electric juicer, or it can be pressed by hand. Before you discard the seeds after juicing, consider keeping them as a salad topping or a snack on their own. To prepare the pomegranate juice, take two large, ripe pomegranates and cut into quarters. Scrape the seeds and flesh from the peels and deposit into the juicer, and press. If you prefer to keep some of the seeds, remove them before adding the fruit to the press. Serve without any added sugar or salt and note that serving sizes may vary depending on the fruit's size and portion.

Pomegranate juice is a powerful support for the kidneys and especially effective while on dialysis. Studies support some benefits due to the high level of antioxidants, preventing the development of free radicals that contribute to infections and other complications such as inflammation, causing the overall condition to worsen if left untreated. It's a delicious juice that can easily fit into a daily diet during any meal. Consuming pomegranate juice is also a good way to prevent kidney disease and high blood pressure while supporting overall immune health. (WebMD Health News, 2010)

APPLE CIDER VINEGAR

In recent years, apple cider vinegar has become a popular option for natural health remedies as a detoxifying agent and a way to support weight loss and overall health. While it's not considered a drink on its own, apple cider vinegar is often diluted to be consumed in water or juice, or taken in a capsule form, if not by spoon. One of the top benefits of regularly taking just one or two tablespoons each day is weight loss. Apple cider vinegar also improves hair and skin appearance and can help regulate insulin and decrease blood sugar. These benefits have the combined effect of supporting the kidneys and making their job a lot easier.

APPLE CIDER

A flavorful beverage hot or cold, apple cider is an excellent drink for kidney health. It's less intense than apple cider vinegar and often enjoyed as a warm beverage during the year's colder months. High in vitamin C, apple cider offers a good boost in antioxidants to the body, supporting the kidneys. It's a good alternative to hot chocolate and other hot drinks flavored with sugar and additives. To sweeten apple cider, add a dash of raw sugar, honey, or maple syrup.

CRANBERRY JUICE

Cranberry juice is an excellent diuretic and is often recommended to prevent and treat bladder infection and related difficulties. It acts as a diuretic because it helps the body flush out excess sodium while reducing water retention, much like water pills. It's a good source of vitamin C and fiber and can aid the kidneys in their function. Cranberry juice is naturally sweet and tangy, which makes it easy to enjoy. Cranberries also offer other benefits linked to kidney health, including fighting infection, improving urinary tract function, and improving digestion.

LEMON JUICE

Lemonade is often sweetened as the preferred lemon-based drink, though it's best to avoid sugary versions and add fresh lemon juice to various drinks or water to boost the vitamin C content. Adding one or two slices of lemon to a glass of iced or sparkling water is a good way to add a splash of flavor without sugar or artificial sweeteners.

LIME JUICE

Like freshly squeezed lemon juice, lime can be used similarly as an added enhancement to water or another juice. Both limes and lemons are high in antioxidants and fiber, making them ideal for your overall health.

MINT AND LEMON WITH CRUSHED ICE

A thirst-quenching and refreshing drink, combining fresh mint leaves with squeezed lime and lemon juice, is a good way to satisfy your thirst and get many vitamins at once. Mint is easy to grow and harvest, or it can be found in fresh or dried varieties at your local market or grocery store. The leaves can be added whole, with ice cubes, sliced, and blended with lemon or lime juice and ice.

GRAPEFRUIT JUICE

Pink grapefruit is often chosen instead of the white variety due to its sweeter taste, though either option is excellent. Enjoyed as is or pressed into a juice, grapefruit can decrease the likelihood of kidney stone development while providing your body with vitamin C and fiber.

CARROT JUICE

The beta carotene in carrots is widely recognized as being good for your vision and eye health, but this is also the case when it comes to your renal function. Carrots offer a boost to the detoxification process, giving kidneys the added push, they need without causing any negative side effects. Carrots are also a delicious part of many meals, though the taste is stronger when consumed raw as a juice. For this reason, carrots are often juiced along with a few slices of apple or orange.

WINE

In moderation and small amounts, wine may offer some improvements in mild or moderate kidney disease cases. If you have a more advanced renal failure stage, you might want to avoid alcohol altogether or seek a medical opinion first. When selecting a wine, choose a dry, low-sugar option that will not increase glucose or blood sugar levels. Keep the drink size small and enjoy on occasion with a meal. Drink plenty of water after, like wine, like other alcoholic beverages, can deplete the body's water and require hydration. If you drink more than two glasses, be sure to increase your water intake and enjoy a small, healthy snack.

WATER

The best drink of all for any organs, including the kidneys, is water. Filtered and oxidized water options are often preferred in areas where there are high levels of contamination and concerns about toxicity, which, in large amounts, can harm the kidneys. If you are fortunate to have excellent quality water sources, make the most of it, and drink water often.

CHAPTER 10

BEST ADVICE TO AVOID DIALYSIS

E ven though it's frightening to be diagnosed with chronic kidney disease (CKD), if you discover in the beginning periods of the symptoms, there are steps you can take to keep away from dialysis. If you work intimately with your PCP, the odds are high you can, in any case, appreciate a refreshing personal satisfaction with kidney disease. Following excellent health practices and evading dialysis, remaining at work, and understanding social exercises are ways individuals can feel responsible for their condition. Notwithstanding doing everything physically and medicinally conceivable to maintain a strategic distance from dialysis, having an occupation with medical coverage gives security that pay, and medical advantages will be accessible. Here are portions of the means to take to maintain a strategic distance from the beginning of dialysis;

EAT RIGHT AND LOSE EXCESS WEIGHT

Consistently make sure to know about serving sizes. It's what you eat that includes calories, yet also how much. As you get in shape, make sure to follow a smart dieting plan that consists of an assortment of Nourishments.

EXERCISE CONSISTENTLY

Most dialysis patients accept they can't work out. In all certainty, most dialysis patients can work out. Numerous renal patients depict regular exercise as the principal action that made them feel "normal" again after beginning dialysis medications. Regardless of whether it is just for a brief timeframe every day, movement allows the patient with persistent kidney disease to feel good, more grounded, and more responsible for their health. Medicinal experts working in renal recovery have demonstrated that an ordinary exercise program, anyway restricted, not just upgrades an individual's potential for physical action, also improves the general personal satisfaction for individuals on dialysis. Exercise can also help the kidney symptoms patient recover the function to perform activities they were delighted in before being analyzed.

TRY NOT TO SMOKE

In case you smoke, there is, in all likelihood, no other choice you can make to help your health more than stopping. While an on-going examination found that smokers lose ten years of life expectancy at any rate than people who never smoked, in like manner found that people who halted by age 40 reduce their risk of smoking-related death by 90 rates.

BE CAUTIOUS OF YOUR GLUCOSE LEVELS

For good preventive health, cut back on soda pop, treats, and sugary baked goods, which can make glucose rise. If you have diabetes, this can hurt your heart, kidneys, eyes, and nerves after some time. Directing glucose is one of seven estimations for heart health, according to the American Heart Association. These equal estimations make it less slanted to be resolved to have malignancy.

FATTY INTAKE

the body needs calories for daily activities and looks after temperature, development, and sufficient body weight. Calories are provided mostly via starches and fats. The standard caloric necessity of CKD patients is 35 - 40 kcal/kg body weight every day. If caloric intake is insufficient, the body uses protein to get calories. This breakdown of protein can prompt severe impacts, for example, lack of healthy sustenance and a more prominent composition of waste items. It is along these lines basic to give a sufficient measure of calories to CKD patients. It is essential to ascertain the caloric necessity indicated by a patient's optimal body weight and not current weight.

STARCHES

These are the essential source of calories for the body. Starches are found in wheat, grains, rice, potatoes, organic products, sugar, nectar, treats, cakes, desserts, and beverages. People with diabetes and fat patients need to confine the measure of starches. It is ideal to use complex sugars from grains like entire wheat and unpolished rice, giving fiber. These should form a large segment of the sugars in the eating regimen. All other basic sugar-containing substances should form not over 20% of the total starch consumption, particularly in diabetic patients. Non-diabetic patients may exchange calories from protein with starches as natural products, pies, cakes, treats, jam, or nectar as long as sweets with chocolate, nuts, or bananas are restricted.

Unsaturated or great fats like olive oil, nut oil, canola oil, safflower oil, sunflower oil, fish, and nuts are superior to saturated or "terrible" fats, for example, red meat, poultry, whole milk, margarine, ghee, cheese, coconut, and grease. Patients with CKD ought to diminish their intake of immersed fats and cholesterol, as these can cause heart disease. Excessive omega-6 polyunsaturated fats (PUFA) and an extremely high omega-6/omega-3 proportion are unsafe, while low omega-6/omega-3 balance applies valuable impacts. Blends of vegetable oil, as opposed to single oil use, will accomplish this reason. Trans fat-containing substances like potato chips, doughnuts, financially arranged treats, and cakes are potentially hurtful and should be avoided.

LIMIT PROTEIN INTAKE

Protein is fundamental for the fix and upkeep of body tissues. It additionally helps in the mending of wounds and battling against disease. Protein confinement (< 0.8 gm/kg body weight/day) is prescribed for CKD patients not on dialysis to diminish the pace of decreased kidney function and defer the requirement for dialysis and kidney transplantation. Serious protein restriction should be kept away from anyway, given the danger of lack of healthy sustenance. Poor craving is normal in CKD patients. Poor hunger and severe protein restriction together can prompt poor sustenance, weight reduction, absence of vitality, and decrease in body opposition, which increment the danger of death. The consumption of protein enhancements and medications, like creatine utilized for muscle advancement, is best kept away from except if affirmed by a physician or dietician. Protein intake should be expanded to 1.0 – 1.2 gm./kg body weight/day to supplant the proteins lost during the methodology when a patient is on dialysis.

FLUID INTAKE

The kidneys play a significant role in maintaining the amount of water in the body by expelling excess fluid as urine. In patients with CKD, as the kidney function exacerbates, the volume of urine generally reduces. Decreased urine yield prompts fluid maintenance in the body, causing puffiness of the face, growing of the legs and hands, and hypertension. The gathering of fluid in the lungs (a condition called pneumonic blockage or edema) causes shortness of breath and trouble in relaxing. If this isn't controlled, it tends to be hazardous. Excess water in the body is called fluid over-burden. Leg growing (edema), ascites (aggregation of fluid in the stomach pit), the brevity of breath, and weight gain in a brief period are the pieces of information that suggest fluid over-burden.

CHAPTER 11

30 DAY MEAL PLAN

The right approach to a healthy diet is getting a balanced proportion of all necessary nutrients. Balanced diets are not meant for people with healthy kidneys alone. It is possible to get meals having all the vital body requirements even when you are on a specific nutrient restriction therapy. A balanced renal-healthy meal should have the right proportion of calories, proteins, vegetables, fruits, and water. As you know, they have their specific roles in ensuring that the kidneys remain healthy.

Meal planning involves including these in a single serving of food. The point of emphasis is that food should be enjoyed, even when you may have to let go of some things. There are essentials to successful meal planning. The following are some generally useful tips:

- Have an objective. Why are you planning your meals? In this case, the goal is to have healthier kidneys. Your overall aim may be broken down into measurable aims to assess how you are doing.
- A handy knowledge of what you need. Equip yourself with the pros and cons of the renal diet so that there are no blurred lines.
- Although you may not need to make regular visits to a dietician at this stage, it will be good to have one look over the meal plan. There may need to make additions or subtractions. Emphasis is on individuality in this plan. Therefore, your dietician may need to go over the plan to be sure it is tailored to meet your specific needs. If you don't have one, consult your doctor.
- Be open-minded. There may be restrictions that make you unhappy but bear in mind that this is not for nothing. The little inconvenience can't be compared with the healthy results.

- Be flexible with your plans. It is good to have interchangeable alternatives when planning meals.
- Work with your budget. What is the essence of organizing what you will eat if you end up stressing yourself over the money? Work on a diet based on your financial capability.

Meal planning is not without its benefits.

- It helps to maximize time, resources, and money.

With meal planning, you can reason thoroughly on the menu, putting whatever is available into good use, and minimizing wastage. There is no rush, and you are relaxed. You also end up saving yourself some energy because everything is organized.

- Planning your meals puts a personal touch on it.

It gives you gratification and a sense of belonging. It does feel good to do something meaningful for oneself, especially when the news of chronic kidney disease is taking its toll on your emotions.

- Helps in creating colorful, delicious, and appealing meals.

Eating goes beyond just having to put something in the stomach. It should come with a satisfaction that is more than just killing your hunger.

- It helps in adherence.

Dieting needs discipline. When you think about the food or edibles you need to do without, you may get tempted to ditch everything and throw caution to the wind.

- It takes care of the craving.

You may feel the urge to binge on some forbidden foods at times. However, with a handy meal menu from adequate planning, it becomes easier to curb it and go with what you have. Sometimes, excessive hunger is what leads to bingeing. When you feel hungry, and there is nothing to satisfy it, your body changes, secreting hormones that heighten the sense of hunger so much that you will eat the available food if there is no control.

- Meal planning curbs extravagant spending during shopping.

You know what you need. Therefore, your trip to the grocery yields only the essentials and unnecessary stuff, something most people find difficult to do.

DAYS	BREAKFAST	LUNCH	DINNER
1	Apple Cherry Breakfast Risotto	Lettuce Wraps with Chicken	Cilantro-Lime Flounder
2	Creamy Keto Cucumber Salad	Peanut Butter and Jelly Grilled Sandwich	Minced Beef Samosa
3	Tasty Beef and Liver Burger	Crispy Lemon Chicken	Green Tuna Salad
4	Shredded Chicken Chili	Grilled Corn on the Cob	Meatloaf Sandwiches
5	Hot Fruit Salad	Cucumber Sandwich	Roasted Chicken and Vegetables
6	Bacon and Cheese Quiche	Ciabatta Rolls with Chicken Pesto	Salmon and Green Beans
7	Egg and Broccoli Casserole	Mexican Steak Tacos	Mango Cheesecake Smoothie
8	Berries and Cream Breakfast Cake	Marinated Shrimp Pasta Salad	Cucumber and Dill Cold Soup
9	Spinach Goat Cheese & Chorizo Omelet	Pizza Pitas	Herb-Crusted Baked Haddock
10	Rice Milk	Beer Pork Ribs	Pizza Pitas
11	Mexican Style Burritos	Grilled Shrimp with Cucumber Lime Salsa	Baked Macaroni & Cheese
12	Blueberry Muffins	Eggplant Casserole	Beef Enchiladas
13	Berry Chia with Yogurt	Turkey Pinwheels	Eggplant Casserole
14	Cheesy Scrambled Egg with Fresh Herbs	Asparagus Fried Rice	Chicken Stew
15	Egg and Veggie Muffins	Shrimp Scampi Linguine	Simple Cabbage Soup
16	Turkey and Spinach Scramble	Vegetable Minestrone	Cilantro and Chili Infused Swordfish

17	Bucket wheat and Grapefruit Porridge	Thai Fish Soup	Feta Bean Salad
18	Apple Pie	Chicken Tacos	Chicken and Savory Rice
19	Eggplant Chicken Sandwich	Curried Carrot and Beet Soup	Chicken and Broccoli Casserole
20	Panzanella Salad	Chicken and Broccoli Casserole	Couscous with Veggies
21	Chorizo Bowl with Corn	Vegetable Biryani	Pork Souvlaki
22	Eggs in Tomato Rings	Simple Chicken and Rice Soup	Cauliflower Rice
23	Arugula Eggs with Chili Peppers	Tuna Twist	Meatball Soup
24	Hot Cocoa	Mexican Chorizo Sausage	Sunny Pineapple Smoothie
25	Bulgur, Couscous and Bucket wheat Cereal	Pesto Pasta Salad	Mexican Chorizo Sausage
26	Poached Asparagus and Egg	Tuna Twist	Creamy Shells with Peas and Bacon
27	Spinach and Ham Frittata	Grilled Onion and Pepper Jack Grilled Cheese Sandwich	Double-Boiled Stewed Potatoes
28	Blueberry Smoothie	Shrimp Quesadilla	Barley Blueberry Avocado Salad
29	Egg Drop Soup	Spicy Mushroom Stir-Fry	Taco Soup
30	Hot Fruit Salad	Pizza with Chicken and Pesto	Spicy Mushroom Stir-Fry

CHAPTER 12

BREAKFAST RECIPES

1 TASTY BEEF AND LIVER BURGER

Preparation Time: 5 minutes

Cooking Time: 5 minutes

Servings: 4

INGREDIENTS:

- ½ medium red onion, peeled
- 1 tsp sea salt
- 1 tsp poultry seasoning
- ¼ pound chicken livers
- pounds beef
- 1 ½ tsp coriander
- 1 tsp ground black pepper

DIRECTIONS:

1. Add the onion and chicken liver to a food processor and process until blended.
2. Put in the ground beef and all the ingredients.
3. Blend for about 1 minute until the ingredients combined thoroughly.
4. Mold the mixture into four-inch wide patties.
5. Broil patties until it is done to your desired taste.
6. Serve on a lettuce wrap or hamburger and enjoy it.

NUTRITION:

Calories: 220
Fat: 4g
Protein: 23g
Sodium: 78mg
Potassium: 344.7mg
Phosphorus: 461mg

2 CREAMY KETO CUCUMBER SALAD

Preparation Time: 5 minutes

Cooking Time: 5 minutes

Servings: 1

INGREDIENTS:

- 2 tbsp of mayo
- Freshly ground pepper
- 2 tbsp lemon juice
- 1 cucumber about
  220grams, sliced

DIRECTIONS:

1. Combine the mayo, lemon juice, and cucumber strips in a medium bowl
2. Put salt and pepper to taste.
3. Serve and enjoy.

NUTRITION:

Calories: 77
Fat: 5g
Carbs: 6g
Protein: 1g
Sodium: 150mg
Potassium: 99mg
Phosphorus: 17mg

3 SHREDDED CHICKEN CHILI

Preparation Time: 10 minutes

Cooking Time: 25 minutes

Servings: 1

INGREDIENTS:

- 1 tbsp butter
- 1 jalapeno pepper, diced
- 2 oz tomato paste
- ½ tbsp garlic powder
- 10 oz diced tomatoes canned
- Salt and pepper to taste
- 4 chicken breasts, shredded
- 1 tbsp chili powder
- 2 cups chicken broth
- 4 oz cream cheese
- ½ onion, diced
- 1 tbsp cumin

DIRECTIONS:

1. Add chicken breast and water to a sizable pot and bring to a boil for 10 to 12 minutes.
2. Once well cooked, take out of the heat and crumble with two forks.
3. Add butter to a large pot and melt over medium to high heat.
4. Add onion and sauté until tender.
5. Add the chicken broth, chili powder, shredded chicken, garlic powder, cumin, and jalapeno to the pot and stir well until evenly blended.
6. Cook over medium to low heat and cover with lid for 10 minutes.
7. Chop cream cheese into 1-inch small strips.

8. Remove the cover and whisk in the cream cheese. Increase the heat to medium-high and keep on whisking until the cream cheese combined thoroughly.
9. Take out of the heat and add salt and pepper to taste. Serve and sprinkle with any desired toppings and enjoy.

NUTRITION:

Calories: 330
Fat: 2.8g
Carbs: 38g
Protein: 38g
Sodium: 716mg
Potassium: 970.7mg
Phosphorus: 421mg

SPINACH, GOAT CHEESE & CHORIZO OMELET

4

Preparation Time: 5 minutes

Cooking Time: 10 minutes

Servings: 1

INGREDIENTS:

- 4 eggs
- 4 ounces chorizo sausage
- ½ tbsp butter
- 1/4 cup salsa Verde (optional)
- 1 tbsp water
- 2 cups baby spinach leaves
-
  2 ounces shredded fresh goat cheese
- Avocado, diced

DIRECTIONS:

1. In a medium-sized frying pan, take out chorizo from the casing and sauté until thoroughly cooked.
2. Meanwhile, add water to a small bowl and beat in the eggs.
3. Remove the chorizo from the skillet with a spoon and keep aside. Clean off the skillet of the remaining oil with a paper towel.
4. Over a moderate flame, melt the butter in the same skillet.
5. Put the cracked eggs in the skillet, and then add the spinach, chorizo, and shredded goat cheese to half of the mixture of the eggs.
6. Heat on low flame for about 3 minutes until a bit dense, then add in the filling and fold over.

7. Cover the skillet with a pot cover and cook on a moderate flame for few minutes until the eggs are evenly cooked.
8. Turn off the stove and allow skillet cover for about 8 minutes while it gets cooked with the extra heat. Serve with slices of avocado and salsa.

NUTRITION:

Calories: 324
Fat: 15.5g
Carbs: 26g
Protein: 21g
Sodium: 389mg
Potassium: 501.3mg
Phosphorus: 238mg

5 APPLE CHERRY BREAKFAST RISOTTO

Preparation Time: 10 minutes

Cooking Time: 15 minutes

Servings: 1

INGREDIENTS:

- 2 large apples, cored and chopped
- 1 ½ cups arborio rice
- ½ cup dried cherries
- 1 ½ tsp cinnamon
- 2 tbsp butter
- ¼ tsp salt
- 1 cup apple juice
- 3 cups of milk

DIRECTIONS:

1. Add butter to the pressure-cooking pot and heat for 2 to 3 minutes.
2. Whisk in the rice, continue heating, and consistently whisk until rice darkens for about 3 to 4 minutes.
3. Put the spices, brown sugar, and apples.
4. Whisk in the juice and milk.
5. Set pressure cooker to high pressure and select 6 minutes cook time and heat.
6. Once the timer beeps, unplug the cooker and use a fast pressure release to release the pressure.
7. Gently remove the lid of the pressure cooker and whisk in dried cherries.
8. Serve hot, and garnish with extra sliced almonds, brown sugar, and milk.

Calories: 258
Fat: 3g
Carbs: 50g
Protein: 10g
Sodium: 227mg
Potassium: 580mg
Phosphorus: 150mg

6 BERRIES AND CREAM BREAKFAST CAKE

Preparation Time: 15 minutes

Cooking Time: 35 minutes

Servings: 1

INGREDIENTS:

- 5 eggs
- ¼ cup of sugar
- 2 tbsp butter, melted
- ¾ cup ricotta cheese
- Sweet yogurt glaze
- Berry Compote
- 2 tsp vanilla extract
- ½ tsp salt
- 1 cup of whole white wheat flour or wheat pastry flour
- 2 tsp baking powder
- ½ cup berry compote

For the sweet yogurt glaze

- ½ tsp vanilla extract
- ¼ cup yogurt
- 1 to 2 tbsp powdered sugar
- 1 tsp milk

DIRECTIONS:

1. First, make ready the berry compote to chill and become thick.
2. For the cake, thoroughly oil a pan with a non-stick cooking spray.
3. Mix the eggs and sugar until blended.

4. Add the ricotta cheese, butter, vanilla, yogurt, and stir until blended.
5. Mix salt, baking powder, and the flour in a separate bowl.
6. Add to the egg mixture. Turn into the prepared pan.
7. With a tablespoon, drop 1/2 cup of berry compote on top of the batter and whisk with a knife.
8. Turn 1 cup of water in the pressure cooker pot and set in the steamer basket. Gently position the pan on the steamer basket.
9. Set the pressure to high. Heat for about 25 minutes.
10. While cooking the cake, prepare the sweet yogurt glaze by mixing the vanilla, yogurt, powdered sugar, and milk.
11. Keep aside. Once cooking is completed, use a normal release to vent pressure for 10 minutes and then release any further pressure.
12. Take out the pan from the pressure cooker. Allow chilling a bit. Loosen the edges of the cake off the pan and lightly pour on a plate.
13. Sprinkle with sweet yogurt glaze and serve hot.

NUTRITION:

Calories: 275
Fat: 13g
Carbs: 36g
Protein: 5g
Sodium: 110.8mg
Potassium: 175.6mg
Phosphorus: 78mg

7 EGG AND BROCCOLI CASSEROLE

Preparation Time: 15 minutes

Cooking Time: 3 hours

Servings: 1

INGREDIENTS:

- ½ tsp salt
- 3 cups frozen, sliced broccoli, thawed and drained
- 6 eggs
- 3 tbsp thinly sliced onion
- 2 cups crumbled cheddar cheese
- ¼ cup butter softened
- 3 cups of cottage cheese
- Extra crumbled cheddar cheese, optional
- 1/3 cup all-purpose flour

DIRECTIONS:

1. Combine all the ingredients in a sizable bowl. Turn into a greased instant pot.
2. Set in the lid and cook on high for 1 hour, then whisk.
3. Lower the heat, place in the lid and cook for an additional 2 hours 30 minutes to 3 hours until a thermometer shows 160 degrees.
4. Unplug the cooker, take out your meal and spread in cheese, and enjoy.

NUTRITION:

Calories: 260
Fat: 13g
Carbs: 10g
Protein: 23g

Sodium: 335mg
Potassium: 161.6mg
Phosphorus: 82.8mg

8 SPINACH AND HAM FRITTATA

Preparation Time: 15 minutes

Cooking Time: 2 – 3 hours

Servings: 1

INGREDIENTS:

- 1 tsp coconut oil
- 8 eggs, whisked
- ½ tsp pepper
- 1 small onion, sliced
- 1 tsp sea salt
- 2 cloves garlic
- 2 cups spinach, diced
- 1 cup ham, sliced
- ½ cup of canned coconut milk

DIRECTIONS:

1. Melt coconut oil in a medium pan.
2. Put onion and garlic and cook until softened.
3. Pour the mixture of the garlic and onion in the instant pot.
4. Add in the ham and spinach.
5. Whisk ingredients until well blended.
6. In a separate bowl, combine coconut milk, whisked egg mixture, salt, pepper, and whisked with a stirrer until well blended.
7. Turn the mixture into the cooking pot and stir well.
8. Set the cooker to low and cook for 4 to 6 hours until the egg is set. You can as well set to high and cook for 2 to 3 hours.
9. Once done, serve warm and enjoy.

Calories: 390
Fat: 24g
Carbs: 6g
Protein: 35g
Sodium: 847mg
Potassium: 145.9mg
Phosphorus: 41mg

9 HOT FRUIT SALAD

Preparation Time: 10 minutes

Cooking Time: 2 – 3 hours

Servings: 1

INGREDIENTS:

- ¾ cups of sugar
- ¼ tsp ground nutmeg
- ¼ cup dried cranberries
- ½ cup butter, melted
- ¼ tsp ground cinnamon
- 1/8 tsp salt
- ½ cup dried apricots, sliced
- 2 (15 1/4-ounce) cans of chopped peaches, drained
- 2 (15 1/4-ounce) cans of diced pears, not drained
- One 23-ounce jar of chunky applesauce

DIRECTIONS:

1. Mix the butter, sugar, nutmeg, cinnamon, and salt in the instant pot.
2. Turn in the rest ingredients.
3. Place in the lid and cook on high until evenly cooked.
4. Allow cooling and then serve.

NUTRITION:

Calories: 152
Fat: 0.1g
Carbs: 39g
Protein: 0.7g
Sodium: 15mg
Potassium: 220.6mg
Phosphorus: 21mg

10 BACON AND CHEESE QUICHE

Preparation Time: 5 minutes

Cooking Time: 4 hours

Servings: 1

INGREDIENTS:

- 1 cup milk
- ¼ tsp salt
- ¼ tsp freshly ground pepper
- 1 box refrigerated pie crusts
- 6 eggs
- 1 cup cooked bacon
- 2 cups crumbled Monterrey jack cheese

DIRECTIONS:

1. Grease 5 to 6-quart slow oval cooker with a cooking spray.
2. Press halves of pie crust 2 inches up the side and halve in the bottom in the cooker, to extend over seams by 1/4 inch.
3. Heat for 1 hour 30 minutes on high.
4. Turn in stirred eggs and bacon over the mixture.
5. Garnish with cheese and seasonings.
6. Heat on low for 2 hours 30 minutes

NUTRITION:

Calories: 524
Fat: 34g
Carbs: 22g
Protein: 25g

Sodium: 826mg
Potassium: 174.8mg
Phosphorus: 287.1mg

11 TURKEY AND SPINACH SCRAMBLE ON MELBA TOAST

Preparation Time: 5 minutes

Cooking Time: 15 minutes

Servings: 2

INGREDIENTS:

- 1 tsp. Extra virgin olive oil
- 1 cup Raw spinach
- ½ clove, minced Garlic
- 1 tsp. grated Nutmeg
- 1 cup Cooked and diced turkey breast
- 4 slices Melba toast
- 1 tsp. Balsamic vinegar

DIRECTIONS:

1. Heat a skillet over medium heat and add oil.
2. Add turkey and heat through for 6 to 8 minutes.
3. Add spinach, garlic, and nutmeg and stir-fry for 6 minutes more.
4. Plate up the Melba toast and top with spinach and turkey scramble.
5. Drizzle with balsamic vinegar and serve.

NUTRITION:

Calories: 301
Fat: 19g
Carb: 12g
Protein: 19g

Sodium: 360mg
Potassium: 269mg
Phosphorus: 215mg

12 CHEESY SCRAMBLED EGGS WITH FRESH HERBS

Preparation Time: 15 minutes

Cooking Time: 10 minutes

Servings: 4

INGREDIENTS:

- 3 Eggs
- 2 Egg whites
- ½ cup Cream cheese
- ¼ cup Unsweetened rice milk
-
  1 tbsp. green part only Chopped scallion
- 1 tbsp. Chopped fresh tarragon
- 2 tbsps. Unsalted butter
- Ground black pepper to taste

DIRECTIONS:

1. Whisk the eggs, egg whites, cream cheese, rice milk, scallions, and tarragon. Mix until smooth.
2. Melt the butter in a skillet.
3. Put egg mixture and cook for 5 minutes or until the eggs are thick and curds creamy.
4. Season with pepper and serve.

NUTRITION:

Calories: 221

Fat: 19g

Carb: 3g

Protein: 8g

Sodium: 193mg

Potassium: 140mg

Phosphorus: 119mg

13 MEXICAN STYLE BURRITOS

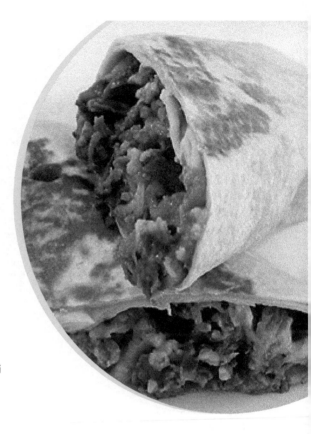

Preparation Time: 5 minutes

Cooking Time: 15 minutes

Servings: 2

INGREDIENTS:

- 1 tbsp. Olive oil
- 2 Corn tortillas
- ¼ cup chopped Red onion
- ¼ cup chopped Red bell peppers
- ½, deseeded and chopped red chili
- 2 Eggs
- 1 lime juice
- 1 tbsp. chopped Cilantro

DIRECTIONS:

1. Place the tortillas in medium heat for 1 to 2 minutes on each side or until lightly toasted.
2. Remove and keep the broiler on.
3. Heat the oil in a skillet and sauté onion, chili, and bell peppers for 5 to 6 minutes or until soft.
4. Crack the eggs over the top of the onions and peppers.
5. Place skillet under the broiler for 5 to 6 minutes or until the eggs are cooked.
6. Serve half the eggs and vegetables on top of each tortilla and sprinkle with cilantro and lime juice to serve.

NUTRITION:

Calories: 202
Fat: 13g
Carb: 19g
Protein: 9g

Sodium: 77mg
Potassium: 233mg
Phosphorus: 184mg

14 BULGUR, COUSCOUS, AND BUCKWHEAT CEREAL

Preparation Time: 10 minutes

Cooking Time: 25 minutes

Servings: 4

INGREDIENTS:

2 ¼ cups Water
1 ¼ cups Vanilla rice milk
6 Tbsps. Uncooked bulgur
2 Tbsps. Uncooked whole buckwheat
1 cup Sliced apple
6 Tbsps. Plain uncooked couscous
½ tsp. Ground cinnamon

DIRECTIONS:

1. Heat the water and milk in the saucepan over medium heat. Let it boil.
2. Put the bulgur, buckwheat, and apple.
3. Reduce the heat to low and simmer, occasionally stirring until the bulgur is tender, about 20 to 25 minutes.
4. Remove the saucepan and stir in the couscous and cinnamon—cover for 10 minutes.
5. Put the cereal before serving.

NUTRITION:

Calories: 159
Fat: 1g
Carb: 34g
Protein: 4g

Sodium: 33mg
Potassium: 116m
Phosphorus: 130mg

15 BLUEBERRY MUFFINS

Preparation Time: 15 minutes

Cooking Time: 30 minutes

Servings: 12

INGREDIENTS:

- 2 cups Unsweetened rice milk
- 1 Tbsp. Apple cider vinegar
- 3 ½ cups All-purpose flour
- 1 cup Granulated sugar
- 1 Tbsp. Baking soda substitute
- 1 tsp. Ground cinnamon
- ½ tsp. Ground nutmeg
- Pinch ground ginger
- ½ cup Canola oil
- 2 Tbsps. Pure vanilla extract
- 2 ½ cups Fresh blueberries

DIRECTIONS:

1. Preheat the oven to 375F.
2. Prepare a muffin pan and set aside.
3. Stir together the rice milk and vinegar in a small bowl. Set aside for 10 minutes.
4. In a large bowl, stir together the sugar, flour, baking soda, cinnamon, nutmeg, and ginger until well mixed.
5. Add oil and vanilla to the milk and mix.
6. Put milk mixture to dry ingredients and stir well to combine.
7. Put the blueberries and spoon the muffin batter evenly into the cups.
8. Bake the muffins for 25 to 30 minutes or until golden and a toothpick inserted comes out clean.
9. Cool for 15 minutes and serve.

Calories: 331
Fat: 11g
Carb: 52g
Protein: 6g
Sodium: 35mg
Potassium: 89mg
Phosphorus: 90mg

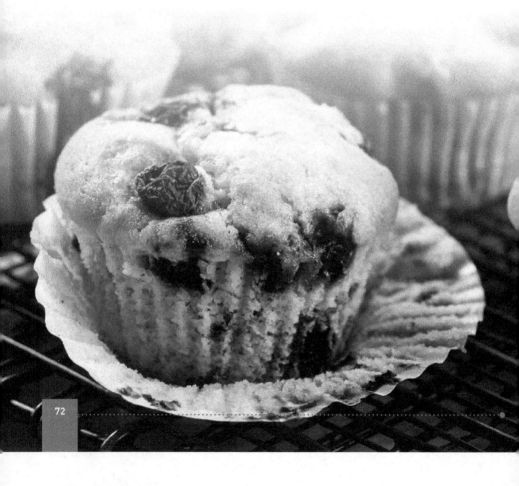

16 BUCKWHEAT AND GRAPEFRUIT PORRIDGE

Preparation Time: 5 minutes

Cooking Time: 20 minutes

Servings: 2

INGREDIENTS:

- ½ cup Buckwheat
- ¼ chopped Grapefruit
- 1 Tbsp. Honey
- 1 ½ cups Almond milk
- 2 cups Water

DIRECTIONS:

1. Let the water boil on the stove. Add the buckwheat and place the lid on the pan.
2. Lower heat slightly and simmer for 7 to 10 minutes, checking to ensure water does not dry out.
3. When most of the water is absorbed, remove, and set aside for 5 minutes.
4. Drain any excess water from the pan and stir in almond milk, heating through for 5 minutes.
5. Add the honey and grapefruit.
6. Serve.

NUTRITION:

Calories: 231
Fat: 4g
Carb: 43g
Protein: 13g
Sodium: 135mg
Potassium: 370mg
Phosphorus: 165mg

EGG AND VEGGIE MUFFINS

Preparation Time: 15 minutes

Cooking Time: 20 minutes

Servings: 4

INGREDIENTS:

- · 4 Eggs
- · 2 Tbsp. Unsweetened rice milk
- · ½ chopped Sweet onion
- · ½ chopped Red bell pepper
- · Pinch red pepper flakes
- · Pinch ground black pepper

DIRECTIONS:

1. Preheat the oven to 350F.
2. Spray 4 muffin pans with cooking spray. Set aside.
3. Whisk the milk, eggs, onion, red pepper, parsley, red pepper flakes, and black pepper until mixed.
4. Pour the egg mixture into prepared muffin pans.
5. Bake until the muffins are puffed and golden, about 18 to 20 minutes. Serve.

NUTRITION:

Calories: 84
Fat: 5g
Carb: 3g
Protein: 7g
Sodium: 75mg
Potassium: 117mg
Phosphorus: 110mg

18 BERRY CHIA WITH YOGURT

Preparation Time: 35 minutes

Cooking Time: 5 minutes

Servings:4

INGREDIENTS:

- ½ cup chia seeds, dried
- 2 cup Plain yogurt
- 1/3 cup strawberries, chopped
- ¼ cup blackberries
- ¼ cup raspberries
- 4 teaspoons Splenda

DIRECTIONS:

1. Mix up together Plain yogurt with Splenda, and chia seeds.
2. Transfer the mixture into the serving ramekins (jars) and leave for 35 minutes.
3. After this, add blackberries, raspberries, and strawberries. Mix up the meal well.
4. Serve it immediately or store it in the fridge for up to 2 days.

NUTRITION:

Calories: 150
Fat: 5g
Carbs: 19g
Protein: 6.8g
Sodium: 65mg
Potassium: 226mg
Phosphorus: 75mg

19 ARUGULA EGGS WITH CHILI PEPPERS

Preparation Time: 7 minutes

Cooking Time: 10 minutes

Servings: 4

INGREDIENTS:

- 2 cups arugula, chopped
- 3 eggs, beaten
- ½ chili pepper, chopped
- 1 tablespoon butter
- 1 oz Parmesan, grated

DIRECTIONS:

1. Toss butter in the skillet and melt it.
2. Add arugula and sauté it over medium heat for 5 minutes. Stir it from time to time.
3. Meanwhile, mix up together Parmesan, chili pepper, and eggs.
4. Pour the egg mixture over the arugula and scramble well.
5. Cook for 5 minutes more over medium heat.

NUTRITION:

Calories: 218
Fat: 15g
Carbs: 2.8g
Protein: 17g
Sodium: 656mg
Potassium: 243mg
Phosphorus: 310mg

20 EGGPLANT CHICKEN SANDWICH

Preparation Time: 10 minutes

Cooking Time: 15 minutes

Servings: 2

INGREDIENTS:

- 1 eggplant, trimmed
- 10 oz chicken fillet
- 1 teaspoon Plain yogurt
- ½ teaspoon minced garlic
- 1 tablespoon fresh cilantro, chopped
- 2 lettuce leaves
- 1 teaspoon olive oil
- ½ teaspoon salt
- ½ teaspoon chili pepper
- 1 teaspoon butter

DIRECTIONS:

1. Slice the eggplant lengthwise into 4 slices.
2. Rub the eggplant slices with minced garlic and brush with olive oil.
3. Grill the eggplant slices on the preheated to 375F grill for 3 minutes from each side.
4. Meanwhile, rub the chicken fillet with salt and chili pepper.
5. Place it in the skillet and add butter.
6. Roast the chicken for 6 minutes from each side over medium-high heat.
7. Cool the cooked eggplants gently and spread one side of them with Plain yogurt.
8. Add lettuce leaves and chopped fresh cilantro.
9. After this, slice the cooked chicken fillet and add over the lettuce.
10. Cover it with the remaining sliced eggplant to get the sandwich shape. Pin the sandwich with the toothpick if needed.

Calories: 276
Fat: 11g
Carbs: 41g
Protein: 13.8g
Sodium: 775mg
Potassium: 532mg
Phosphorus: 187mg

21 EGGS IN TOMATO RINGS

Preparation Time: 8 minutes

Cooking Time: 5 minutes

Servings: 2

INGREDIENTS:

- 1 tomato
- 2 eggs
- ¼ teaspoon chili flakes
- ¾ teaspoon salt
- ½ teaspoon butter

DIRECTIONS:

1. Trim the tomato and slice it into 2 rings.
2. Remove the tomato flesh.
3. Toss butter in the skillet and melt it.
4. Then arrange the tomato rings.
5. Crack the eggs in the tomato rings. Sprinkle them with salt and chili flakes.
6. Cook the eggs for 4 minutes over medium heat with the closed lid.
7. Transfer the cooked eggs into the serving plates with the help of the spatula.

NUTRITION:

Calories: 237
Fat: 16g
Carbs: 7g
Protein: 16g
Sodium: 427mg
Potassium: 391.5mg
Phosphorus: 291mg

22 CHORIZO BOWL WITH CORN

Preparation Time: 10 minutes

Cooking Time: 15 minutes

Servings: 4

INGREDIENTS:

- 9 oz chorizo
- 1 tablespoon almond butter
- ½ cup corn kernels
- 1 tomato, chopped
- ¾ cup heavy cream
- 1 teaspoon butter
- ¼ teaspoon chili pepper
- 1 tablespoon dill, chopped

DIRECTIONS:

1. Chop the chorizo and place it in the skillet.
2. Add almond butter and chili pepper.
3. Roast the chorizo for 3 minutes.
4. After this, add tomato and corn kernels.
5. Add butter and chopped the dill. Mix up the mixture well—Cook for 2 minutes.
6. Close the lid and simmer for 10 minutes over low heat.
7. Transfer the cooked meal into the serving bowls.

NUTRITION:

Calories: 286
Fat: 15g
Carbs: 26g
Protein: 13g

Sodium: 228mg
Potassium: 255mg
Phosphorus: 293mg

23 PANZANELLA SALAD

Preparation Time: 10 minutes

Cooking Time: 5 minutes

Servings: 4

INGREDIENTS:

- 3 tomatoes, chopped
- 2 cucumbers, chopped
- 1 red onion, sliced
- 2 red bell peppers, chopped
- ¼ cup fresh cilantro, chopped
- 1 tablespoon capers
- 1 oz whole-grain bread, chopped
- 1 tablespoon canola oil
- ½ teaspoon minced garlic
- 1 tablespoon Dijon mustard
- 1 teaspoon olive oil
- 1 teaspoon lime juice

DIRECTIONS:

1. Pour canola oil into the skillet and bring it to boil.
2. Add chopped bread and roast it until crunchy (3-5 minutes).
3. Meanwhile, in the salad bowl, combine sliced red onion, cucumbers, tomatoes, bell peppers, cilantro, capers, and mix up gently.
4. Make the dressing: mix up together lime juice, olive oil, Dijon mustard, and minced garlic.
5. Put the dressing over the salad and stir it directly before serving.

NUTRITION:

Calories: 224.3
Fat: 10g
Carbs: 26g

Protein: 6.6g
Sodium: 401mg

Potassium: 324.9mg
Phosphorus: 84mg

24 POACHED ASPARAGUS AND EGG

Preparation time: 3 minutes

Cooking Time: 15 minutes

Servings: 1

INGREDIENTS:

- 1 egg
- 4 spears asparagus
- Water

DIRECTIONS:

1. Half-fill a deep saucepan with water set over high heat. Let the water come to a boil.
2. Dip asparagus spears in water. Cook until they turn a shade brighter, about 3 minutes. Remove from saucepan and drain on paper towels. Keep warm—lightly season before serving.
3. Use a slotted spoon to lower the egg into boiling water gently.
4. Cook for only 4 minutes. Remove from pan immediately. Place on egg holder.
5. Slice off the top. The egg should still be fluid inside.
6. Place asparagus spears on a small plate and serve egg on the side.
7. Dip asparagus into the egg and eat while warm.

NUTRITION:

Calories: 178
Fat: 13g
Carbs: 1g
Protein: 7.72g

Calories 178
Sodium: 71mg
Potassium: 203mg
Phosphorus: 124mg

25 EGG DROP SOUP

Preparation Time: 5 minutes

Cooking Time: 10 minutes

Servings:4

INGREDIENTS:

- ¼ cup minced fresh chives
- 4 cups unsalted vegetable stock
- 4 whisked eggs

DIRECTIONS:

1. Pour unsalted vegetable stock into the oven set over high heat. Bring to a boil. Lower heat.
2. Pour in the eggs. Stir until ribbons form into the soup.
3. Turn off the heat immediately. The residual heat will cook eggs through.
4. Cool slightly before ladling the desired amount into individual bowls. Garnish with a pinch of parsley, if using.
5. Serve immediately.

NUTRITION:

Calories: 73
Fat: 3g
Carbs: 1g
Protein: 7g
Sodium: 891mg
Potassium: 53mg
Phosphorus: 36mg

CONCLUSION

When you have chronic kidney disease, it is incredibly important to focus on promoting healthy lifestyle factors. You can't just take some medicine and get better. Instead, you have to prioritize eating a low-protein diet with the correct proportions of nutrients, exercising to maintain healthy muscles and organs, and sleeping well so that your body has the strength to function to the best of its ability. In one study on chronic kidney disease, it was found that patients who eat a healthy diet, stay physically active, maintain healthy body weight, and don't smoke can increase their longevity greatly. The participants who met all of these healthy lifestyle qualities reduced their risks of dying from the disease by sixty-eight percent compared to those who don't follow these lifestyle choices.

These same lifestyle factors have also long been shown to greatly affect heart health and diabetes, in which two-thirds of the population with chronic kidney disease also have. It is important because if your diabetes or heart health is not under control, it will put more pressure on your kidneys and increase your fatality risk. On the other hand, if you treat these conditions through a healthy lifestyle, you can greatly improve your diabetes or heart health and kidney health. Overall, you can only benefit from focusing on improving your lifestyle.

Suppose you don't yet have chronic kidney disease, but you or a family member are at risk of developing the condition. In that case, you can reduce your risk and potentially prevent yourself from developing the disease by making healthy lifestyle changes. Remember, you are more likely to develop kidney disease if you have a family history, diabetes, heart disease, or high blood pressure.

By managing the conditions associated with kidney diseases, such as diabetes and high blood pressure, you can benefit your kidney health and the health of your entire body and mind.

You can take to improving your kidney health is managing your blood pressure. Most people only think about the effect blood pressure has on the heart, but it also affects other organs, such as your kidneys. When blood pressure is chronically high, it causes damage to the kidneys. Therefore, you should maintain blood pressure at the goal set by your physician.

When you experience long-term stress, it greatly affects your health. Not only does stress often increase poor life choices, such as smoking, drinking, irregular sleep, and an unhealthy diet. But, chronically high stress increases blood sugar, raises blood pressure, and may lead to depression. You first need to prioritize a healthy lifestyle overall to manage your stress. Exercise, eating well, sleep, and other healthy lifestyle factors can all reduce chronic anxiety. However, you may need different methods of stress relief, as well. Try making a list of any calming activities you find helpful, such as listening to music, meditation, yoga, sketching, reading, or whatever else comes to mind. You can then use this list as inspiration when you are anxious. Whenever you find your stress increased, try completing one or two calming tasks from your list.

Excessive body weight causes your kidneys to push harder to complete their work and cause damage over time. Not only that, but excess weight also increases your risk of high blood pressure, high blood sugar, and more. Together, all of these aspects worsen kidney health, making it vital to maintain a healthy body weight to increase kidney health.

Adequate sleep and good sleep quality are important for overall physical and mental health. When you don't sleep well, it can negatively affect you in many ways, such as raising blood pressure and blood glucose. Studies have shown that adults should get seven to eight hours of solid sleep a night.

It is best to try to be active for at least thirty minutes a day. However, you should specifically try to maintain thirty minutes of moderate exercise three to four times a week. Along with moderate exercise, it is good to include some light flexibility-based exercises, which can reduce your risk of injury and make your more difficult exercises easier.

Of course, you should take any prescribed medication your doctor gives you. Whenever you see any of your doctors, make sure they all know every single medication you are taking, whether prescribed or over the counter, as well as supplements. These can affect your health in more ways than you might realize, and a simple over-the-counter supplement could negatively interact with one of your conditions or medications.

Besides giving your doctor a list of your medications, you should also talk to either your doctor or pharmacist before taking any new over-the-counter medications or supplements. These can cause many problems, which might not be listed on the label. For instance, many painkillers can damage the kidneys and should not be taken by anyone with kidney disease or injury.

As you know, diet is also an important aspect of your lifestyle so you can live better and longer.

Lightning Source UK Ltd.
Milton Keynes UK
UKHW020700130521
383647UK00001B/63